Risk assessment : understanding base rates

Copyright © 2016 Health Insights

All rights reserved.
No part of this publication may be reproduced, stored, or transmitted in any form or by any means, electronic, mechanical, photocopied, recorded or otherwise, without prior written consent from Health Insights.

Notice of Disclaimer: The information contained in this publication is based on the experience and opinions of the authors. The authors, Health Insights and Liberty Press will not be held liable for the use or misuse of the information in this publication.

Produced for Health Insights by Liberty Press, Cheshire, England

Acknowledgements: Health Insights is grateful for the contribution of those providing the images which have been used to illustrate this publication.

All *Figures* in this publication were produced by Neil Craven for Health Insights

All *Graphic Images* in this publication are courtesy of Creative Commons. Named authors are as follows: Marco Lachman-Anke; Gerd Altmann; Kai Stachowiak; Steve Bidmead and Ralf Kunze.

Contents

Background	1
Advances in risk assessment	2
What is a 'good' method of risk assessment	3
Understanding the key clinical statistics for actuarial tools	5
Base rates: the 'statistical' problem	7
Base rates: the 'cognitive' problem	23
Summary and key points	25
References and further reading	29

Background

Violence in the UK remains a significant public health issue and there is evidence that front-line clinical staff are at particular risk of assault (RCP 2005). Despite overall reductions in violent crime in the wider general population context, changes in the profile of violent crime maintain high levels of public concern regarding the risk of victimisation (Walker et al 2009). Increasingly, over recent decades, clinicians have been identified as having both a moral and legal obligation to protect third parties from foreseeable harm by their clients. In the US, this expectation has been made explicit in the 1976 Tarasoff ruling by the California Legislature. In the UK, recommendations in the 1983 Mental Health Act and subsequent revisions of this Act imply similar attributions of responsibility.

Whether tied to legislative obligations or not, the ramifications of an incorrect risk assessment in relation to violent behaviour are substantial not only for the individual client and clinician but also for potential victims and for society in the wider context. Violence risk assessment is consequently one of the more fraught decisions a clinician has to engage with. Currently, the most prominent form of risk assessment, accepted in the legal context and assumed as standard practice within NHS forensic and related settings is actuarial risk assessment. Yet there remain significant question marks over both the accuracy of available risk assessment tools (Szmukler 2001) and the ability of clinicians to correctly interpret their outcomes (Alberg et al 2004). This guide aims to clarify the interpretation of actuarial risk assessment, focussing in particular on the relevance of population base rates to the interpretation of risk profiles.

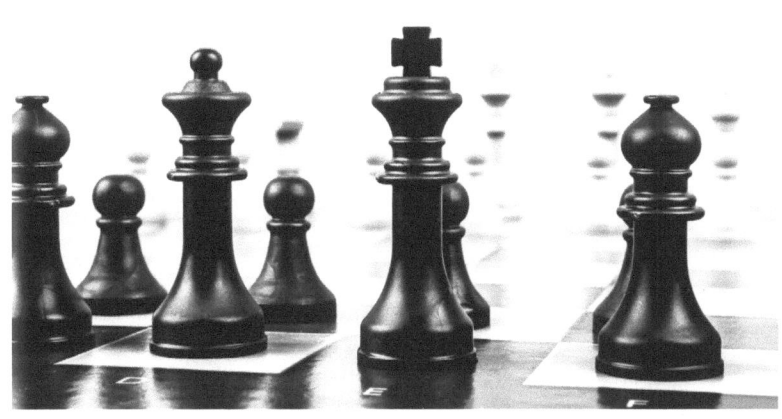

Advances in risk assessment

Historically, violence risk assessment fell solely within the domain of unstructured clinical evaluation and comparatively little attention was paid to the accuracy and outcome of such judgements (Dolan and Doyle 2000). During the 1970s, a spate of research on the outcomes of clinical prediction, stimulated initially by the Baxstrom vs Herald (USA, 1966) ruling[1], questioned the accuracy and broader conceptual validity of clinical assessment. Such assessments have subsequently been identified as having low reliability (both within and between raters and across time); low predictive validity and a lack of conceptual coherence (Monahan & Steadman 1994; Webster et al 1997a; Lidz et al 1993; Mossman 1994). Whilst research does support the contention that clinical judgement is better than chance (Gardner et al 1996) and that taking into account contextual factors (Mulvey & Lidz 1985) and consensus judgements (Fuller & Cowan 1999) improves accuracy, the weight of accumulated evidence undermines confidence in a reliance solely on unsupported clinical judgement in evaluating risk.

During the 1990s, a new generation of semi-structured (e.g. HCR-20, Webster et al 1997b; SVR-20, Boer et al 1997) and structured (e.g. PCL-R, Hare 1991; VRAG, Harris et al 1993) risk assessment tools rose to prominence. These tools explicitly incorporate empirically validated risk items (e.g. past history of child abuse) and are based on and validated using psychometric principles. To date, this generation of risk assessment tool, generally referred to as 'actuarial' risk assessment retains the strongest weight of available research evidence. It has also generated substantial controversy. Risk assessment remains in development, with potential future generations of risk tool focussing on, for example, 'objective' risk assessment contextualised using local clinical knowledge (cf. Shlonsky & Wagner 2005) and classification tree approaches (cf. Monahan et al 2005). Currently, the main focus remains on the 1990's generation of actuarial risk prediction tool.

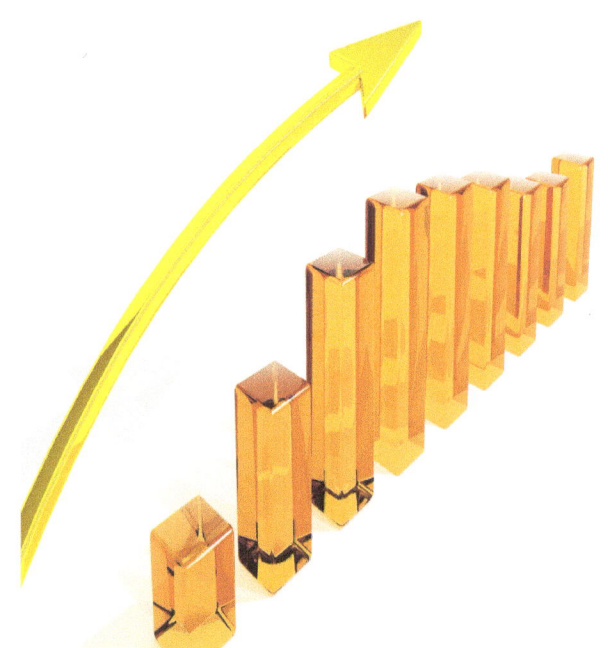

---

1   The Baxstrom vs Herald ruling resulted in the release or transfer of 966 maximum security hospital patients to lower security settings and into the community. A four-year follow-up study by Steadman & Coccoza (1974) identified that despite clinical judgements regarding the severity of risk, in fact only 20% of this cohort were reconvicted, the majority of offences being of a non-violent nature.

What is a 'good' method of risk assessment?

The intuitive appeal of unstructured clinical assessment lies in the fact that, taken at face value, the skills needed to reach a conclusion regarding risk are those which the clinician will naturally have acquired during the normal course of training or practice. Additional arguments put forward to support the continued use of clinical decision making as a risk assessment tool include the flexibility to respond to the needs of the individual client (Snowden 1997), a natural emphasis on risk management (Hart 1998a) and the inherently value-driven nature of determining the costs and benefits of intervening with clients seen to be 'at risk' of violence (Szmukler 2003). These appealing arguments however continue to be undermined by the stark fact that the research evidence to date identifies unstructured clinical prediction as being *wrong* between 70-90% of the time (e.g. Dix 1976; Hall 1988; Kahn and Chambers 1991)

The alternative of actuarial assessment is far from perfect and remains under development (for example, the majority of current tools fail to incorporate dynamic factors and also fail to take into account the interaction between potential offender and potential victim characteristics). Nonetheless, this approach to risk assessment is currently the only approach which stands up in court, literally. So, as Maden (2003) asks, "why all the fuss?". Why does actuarial assessment continue to cause heated debate? Setting aside the normative issues, which are outside the focus of the current guide, one answer is that actuarial tools do not hold a natural appeal for clinicians. In the first place, they are developed within and relate to populations, whilst clinicians are concerned with outcomes for individuals. In the second place, their use requires an ability to intuitively interpret statistical data which may not feature as a key skill in the training given to clinicians.

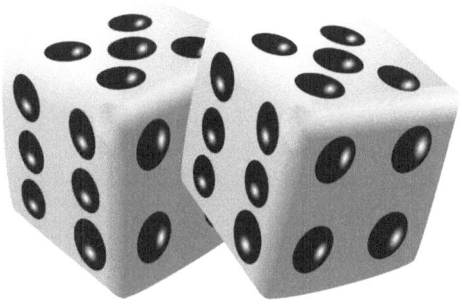

In overcoming such concerns, clinicians are not currently aided by the available information. By way of example, a systematic review (Leitner et al 2006) identified in excess of 200 structured violence risk assessment tools. In evaluating this myriad of tools, the research literature focussed almost exclusively on the psychometric properties of reliability and validity. Considering only the most extensively validated tools, for example (e.g. PCL, Hare 1991; VRAG, Harris et al 1993) only 12% of studies considered the discriminatory power of the actuarial tools, all other evaluations considered *only* reliability and /or validity[1]. Why is this important? In essence, because statistical robustness and clinical robustness are not one and the same thing.

Reliability refers to the ability of a prediction tool to consistently yield the same outcome (between raters; across time; in the same circumstances; for the same individual(s)). Validity refers to the ability of the prediction tool to measure what it claims to measure (e.g. likelihood of repetition, likely severity of future violence). Both are statistical measures of the tool's internal and external coherence. The clinician certainly needs to be aware of these values, but from a clinical perspective their only relevance is that they establish that a tool is worth considering in the first place. Thereafter, they provide little relevant insight. Consider a tool which has both a high reliability (the outcomes it produces are almost always consistent) and a high validity (a strong correlation exists between the scores generated by the tool and violent behaviour in a large reference population of individuals). Now, what does this tell us about the tool's likely performance in clinical practice? The answer is, very little. A risk assessment tool may provide very consistent outcomes, but they may be the wrong outcomes for the client group of interest to the clinician. Equally, a tool may be a valid measure of the risk of violence at the group level, but not be valid at the level of the individual client. So, the key measures of a tool's viability used in the research literature are *not* the measures of greatest interest to the clinician.

What measures are of value to the clinician then? Discriminatory power (the least prominent outcome addressed in the research literature on actuarial tools) gets us closer. Discriminatory power refers to the overall ability of a risk assessment tool to correctly distinguish between groups of individuals not possessing the target characteristic (violent behaviour) and those possessing this characteristic. Closer, but still not ideal. The clinician needs a measure of the tool's function which identifies not an 'average' likely outcome for the classification of a group of individuals, but an estimate of the likely 'success' and 'failure' rate of the tool as it is applied to individual clients. Short of evaluating each tool for every individual client separately, actuarial tools can never achieve this ideal goal (neither, for that matter, can unstructured clinical judgement). However, by taking into account the discrete components which contribute to a tool's discriminatory power it is possible to get within striking distance of this goal. Unfortunately, neither the research literature, nor, in many cases, test manuals tend to cite or interpret these particular statistics for the clinician.

---

1   It is worth noting in addition that many of the evaluative studies also considered only the weakest forms of psychometric evaluation, both statistically and conceptually, for example inter-rater reliability or concurrent validity (the correlation between outcomes from one tool and another tool purporting to measure the same thing).

Understanding the key clinical statistics for actuarial tools

In the research context, the scores generated by actuarial tools are often treated as a continuum of outcomes. In the clinical context, they are more commonly treated as one or more 'cut-off' points which assign a client to a particular category of risk (low, medium, high at most, generally simply 'at risk' or 'not at risk'). This discrete picture of risk is unrealistic in that both risk and protective factors are likely to be cumulative and so the reality of risk *is* closer to a continuum. However, for all practical purposes, placing individuals in a small number of discrete 'risk units' is a necessary evil. This approach makes violence risk assessment analogous to diagnostic choices in the physical health context. For example, on the basis of a cultured sample, an individual may or may not be assigned to a category indicating that they have tuberculosis. This analogy to physical health diagnosis is important, as it helps to identify the key statistics which are of value to the clinician. It also happens to underline the fact that, unlike a diagnosis of tuberculosis, (a pathogen is or is not there), violence risk assessment at some level remains a matter of subjective choice, regardless of the performance of actuarial tools. How much risk is acceptable? In what circumstances and over what length of time?

Briefly put, there are only three key statistics which are fully informative in any clinical model which entails dividing individuals into a small number of discrete categories (cf. Glaros & Kline 1988). These statistics are **sensitivity**, **specificity** and **prevalence**.

In the current context, *sensitivity* can be defined as the specific ability of a risk assessment tool to identify those individuals who will become violent as likely to be violent. *Specificity* can, conversely, be defined as the ability of a risk assessment tool to correctly identify those individuals who will *not* become violent as such. In contrast to these statistics, both of which are features of the assessment tool, *prevalence* is a characteristic of the population and of the extent to which the population being evaluated expresses the trait of interest, in this case violent behaviour. Prevalence then, is defined as the total number of people who actually have been violent in the population at a given time. Prevalence is also termed the 'base rate' of violence in the population[1].

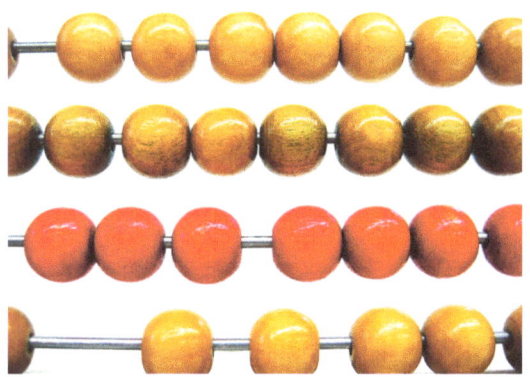

In line with the tuberculosis analogy, these three relatively simple to calculate statistics get the clinician much closer to a useful interpretation of the likely value of an actuarial tool in the practical clinical setting than the more commonly cited psychometric properties of the tool. Conceptually, sensitivity and specificity are clearly what the clinician is most interested in. What is the likelihood that a client who is identified as likely to be violent using the actuarial tool will be violent and what is the, converse, likelihood that he or she will be incorrectly classified as non-violent and vice versa? Sensitivity and specificity then, are the features of an actuarial tool that the clinician should be most closely focussed on in interpreting

---

1 Incidence, which is defined as the number of new cases of a disorder occurring in a population over a specified time period can also be used to represent the population base rate for a disorder.

the likely functionality of the range of actuarial tools available. However, the interpretation of these and related statistics is frequently obscured by a failure to understand the role of prevalence (base rate) in evaluating the outcomes of any evaluation of a particular risk assessment tool. The so called 'base rate problem[2]' (Kahneman & Tversky 1973; Nisbett et al 1976; Bar-Hillel 1980) is actually a composite of three separate issues:

- The dependence of an assessment tool's accuracy on base rates in reference and target populations

- Limitations on predictive values (sensitivity, specificity and related statistics) for rare behaviours

- Cognitive 'misinterpretation' of probabilistic information

The remainder of this guide aims to clarify the interpretation of the above statistics and associated measures of outcome for the evaluation of risk assessment tools and identifies possible errors attributable to a misunderstanding of the role of base rates in interpreting outcomes.

---

[2] Also called the 'problem of prior probabilities'.

Base rates: the 'statistical' problem

Sensitivity, specificity and related statistics are used to evaluate assessment tools with discrete 'cut-off' scores. Estimates for these measures are calculated using contingency tables, also, perhaps disconcertingly, called 'confusion tables'. A contingency table sets out the estimated versus actually observed outcomes for a target behaviour or characteristic. An hypothetical example is set out at Figure 1 below:

Figure 1

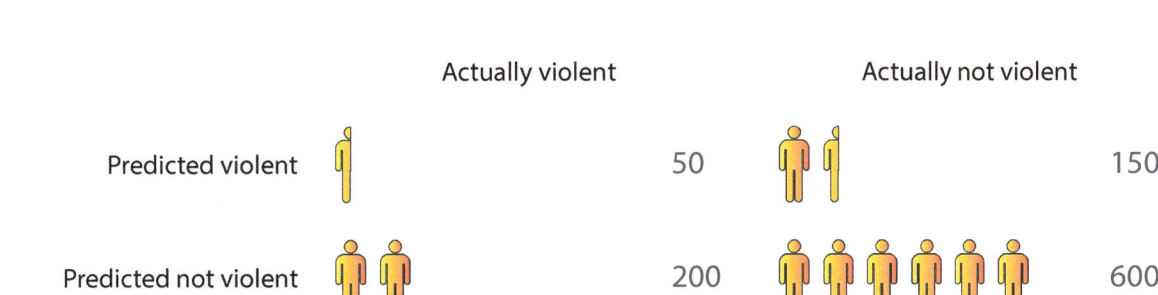

Example of a 2×2 Contingency Table

	Actually violent		Actually not violent	
Predicted violent		50		150
Predicted not violent		200		600

Four main statistics are generally calculated from the type of contingency table set out above. Worked examples are as follows:

- Prevalence (Base rate) = N (actually violent) / Total population
  (250/1000 = 0.25)

- Sensitivity = N (Assessed correctly as violent) / Total N actually violent
  (50/250 = 0.20)

- Specificity = N (Assessed correctly as non-violent) / Total N actually non-violent
  (600/750 = 0.80)

- Accuracy = Total N of correct assessments (violent and non-violent) / Total population
  (650/1000 = 0.65)

A large number of other statistics can be derived from the figures in the above table (cf. Metz 1978), however the four examples above suffice to illustrate the nature of the two 'statistics related' base rate issues in interpreting outcomes.

The first point to note is that risk assessment tools are evaluated in a *reference* population, but utilised in a *target* population (more specifically, applied to an individual client who will be more or less representative of a particular population group). Sensitivity and specificity are values which are directly linked to the characteristics of the reference population in which they were established. Whilst they are attributes of the risk assessment tool for which they were established, they are not immutable attributes of this tool. Suppose the reference population (the population which researchers used to establish the attributes of the risk assessment tool) was comprised solely of male participants, would one expect the sensitivity and specificity of the tool to remain the same for a target population (clients to be assessed by the clinician) comprised solely of female patients? The answer is, only if males and females are relevantly similar with respect to violence. The use of a risk assessment tool is therefore not generalisable from one population to another unless sensitivity and specificity are stable across the two populations. It is an important, but often overlooked, fact that the clinician needs to consider carefully whether the population for which sensitivity and specificity have been established for a particular tool closely matches the client group in which risk assessment is to take place.

One key element of similarity is whether the base rate of violence is equivalent in reference and target populations. However, it is important to understand that measures of sensitivity and specificity are themselves independent of base rate. At first glance, this is unexpected, since the denominators in the equations used to derive sensitivity and specificity are equivalent to base rate and (1-base rate) respectively. Independence is introduced by the fact that the numerators in the equations (Total N actually violent and total N actually non-violent) are empirically derived values. Since these values are empirically established using a reference population, sensitivity and specificity are closely related to the characteristics of that population but, they are not tied either to population size or to the base rate in the reference or clinical populations. So, provided that the clinical population has the same structure as the reference group (e.g. comprises roughly the same proportion of males and females) then, all other things being equal, the sensitivity and specificity of the tool transposed to the clinical setting should remain constant and the clinician should be able to rely on the values obtained in the reference population.

Using the hypothetical figures in the contingency table above to illustrate this point, an assessment tool with a sensitivity of 0.2 which therefore correctly identifies 50 out of 250 people at risk of violence in a reference population of 1000, would be expected to identify 100 out of 500 people in a relevantly similar clinical target population of 2000 (showing independence from population size) and to identify 100 out of 500 people at risk of violence in a population of 1000 with twice the base rate of the reference population (showing independence from base rate). In respect of base rate and population size then, sensitivity and specificity are, conveniently, constants. The caveat regarding the similarity between reference and target populations is an important one to note however. Any statistically significant variance in structure between reference and target populations which is also pertinent to the likelihood of violence renders this constancy null and void. So, reference and target (clinical) populations need to show, for example, the same demographic structure, the same type of violence, the same history of repetition and so on. Weighting procedures can be applied to take into account relevant differences in structure, but these substantially complicate the application of the risk assessment tool in the clinical setting.

In contrast to measures of sensitivity and specificity, measures of overall accuracy are strongly dependent on the base rate of violence in a population. Unfortunately, such measures also have a natural appeal for clinicians. The clinician is equally concerned to avoid false positives (labelling people as violent when they are not) and false negatives (failing to identify people at risk of being violent). Therefore, there is substantive pressure on the clinician to try and identify the overall accuracy of a risk assessment tool. That is, to find a measure of the tool's performance which takes into account both its sensitivity and its specificity. The single number calculated using the equation set out earlier has considerable appeal. Alberg et al (2004) have identified that 'overall accuracy' is a statistic used ubiquitously in clinical trial reports addressing the viability of risk assessment tools. Unfortunately, it seems that its dependence on base rates is generally ignored. Used in this way, the accuracy figure is anything but accurate and can distort both the outcomes for the risk assessment tools being evaluated and the eventual risk assessment of individuals made using these tools.

Looking again at the equation for accuracy, it can be seen that overall accuracy (also called diagnostic accuracy /test efficiency) is the weighted average of a risk assessment tool's sensitivity and specificity. So, given that sensitivity and specificity are independent of population base rate, why is accuracy closely tied to base rate? The answer is that the weighting used to achieve the 'averaging' *is* the base rate. Going back to the contingency table, the equation for accuracy can be re-written as:

$$[(Base\ Rate)(Sensitivity)] + [(1-\ Base\ Rate)(Specificity)]$$

This explicit formulation of the associations between base rate and sensitivity and specificity in the calculation of overall accuracy can be used to identify two situations which give rise to practical problems where accuracy is used to determine the value of a risk assessment tool to the clinician. These particularly critical situations are:

- Divergence between the sensitivity and specificity of a risk assessment tool

- Divergence of the base rate of violence in a population away from 50%

Figure 2 overleaf provides a worked example of how these situations impact on accuracy.

Figure 2

Variations in accuracy as a function of base rate, sensitivity and specificity

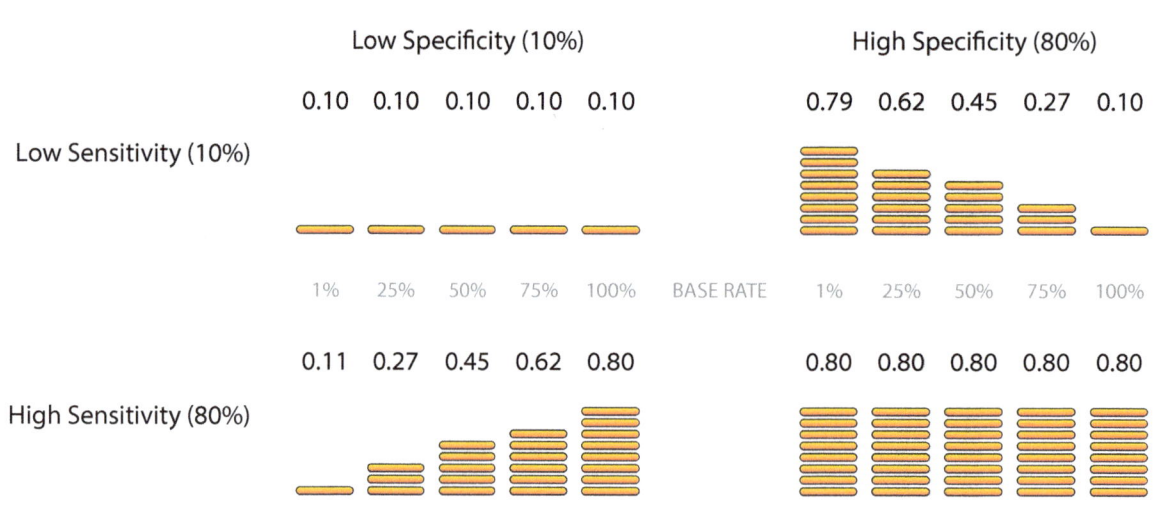

The above Figure deliberately sets out an extreme set of circumstances to illustrate the base rate problem in respect of overall accuracy. Nevertheless, the logic behind the associations represented in the Figure holds in more realistic clinical scenarios. From Figure 2, it can be seen that when there is no divergence between sensitivity and specificity (whether both are high or both are low values) estimated accuracy simply tracks the values for sensitivity and specificity. It tracks these regardless of the population base rate, but in this context it provides no additional information. As values for sensitivity and specificity begin to diverge, it can be seen that as base rates approach low values, estimates of overall accuracy in fact begin to track values for specificity, whilst as base rates approach high values, estimates of overall accuracy begin to track values for sensitivity.

The above characteristics are simply mathematical functions of the equation used to measure overall accuracy. At equivalent values, sensitivity and specificity 'cancel each other out' and accuracy is equivalent to the single value assigned to them. At very low base rates few positive cases are expected in the population, so accuracy necessarily leans towards a measure of the true negatives identified (the people who are not likely to be violent). At high base rates, few negative cases are expected, so accuracy necessarily leans towards a measure of true positives (the people who will be violent). So, the overall accuracy of a risk assessment tool either provides no additional information to sensitivity and specificity taken separately, or it provides information which is biased towards one or other measure.

By way of illustration, consider the 79% accuracy reported in Figure 2 for a 1% base rate, 10% sensitivity and 80% specificity. Taken at face value, 79% overall accuracy for a risk assessment tool sounds excellent. However, this is in fact only a measure of the specificity of the tool (its ability to identify true negatives).

This point often goes unrecognised in the clinical literature and presumably also in clinical practice. Yet, it conclusively undermines the likely clinical value of using overall accuracy as a measure of the efficacy of a risk assessment tool. Consider the following: A new risk assessment tool has been developed which the test developers, correctly, claim is 95% accurate measured against a sample population with a 5% base rate of violence. This sounds ideal, but how does the assessment tool work? Simple, the assessment tool evaluates every individual as being at absolutely no risk of violence! That is, sensitivity is set to 0 and specificity to 1. With a 5% actual population base rate of violence, the assessment tool will necessarily result in an inaccurate assignment on 5% of occasions, but it will, conversely, be 95% accurate at this low base rate. Such an assessment tool would obviously be useless in the clinical setting, yet it is 95% accurate. This demonstrates that overall accuracy is a metric that needs to be approached with considerable caution.

The above discussion aimed to clarify the first 'base rate issue' in respect of interpreting the clinical value of assessment tools. In essence, the point is that it is generally unwise to collapse the more useful measures of sensitivity, specificity and prevalence into the single less valuable measure 'overall accuracy'. Setting aside accuracy then, are we left with any problems if we focus instead simply on specificity and sensitivity? Since these are independent of base rate, surely they can be relied on? The answer here is 'yes… and no'. To illustrate the second type of 'base rate' problem, we can consider one 'real life' case in which base rates are low and there are substantial variations in base rate for different target groups. Cunningham & Reidy (1998) compared the number of serious prison rule violations (homicide; assault with a weapon; striking a prison officer; making a sexual threat) per 100 inmates per year across a range of settings. The resulting base rates for such violations across different target groups are set out below:

- Released Death Row Prisoners: 0.02
- Life Sentence Prisoners: 0.03
- Systemwide: 0.12
- High Security Prisoners: 0.19

These base rates are clearly quite low, but they are real and not at all unusual. Figure 3 overleaf sets out the 'hit rate' of an hypothetical risk assessment tool as measured in the context of the above base rates. The Figure assumes very high (and equal) values for both sensitivity and specificity (80%).

The populations used in the above example are populations in which risk assessment is both common practice and of particular importance given the decisions regarding risk management which may be made as a consequence. The estimates for the base rates of serious infractions are real. The set values for the hypothetical risk assessment tool's sensitivity and specificity are in contrast both implausibly high and also equivalent, giving a 'best case' scenario for the likely efficacy of risk assessment using the hypothetical tool in these real populations.

A risk assessment tool with the very high values of sensitivity and specificity outlined is an implausible beast. Yet, as the Figure demonstrates, even such a strong predictor struggles in a situation where the behaviour to be predicted is rare. It should again be noted that sensitivity and specificity are intrinsically independent of base rate, so the issue explored here is not equivalent to the problem outlined above in respect of overall accuracy. Rather, it is a function of the intrinsic difficulty of predicting rare events.

Figure 3

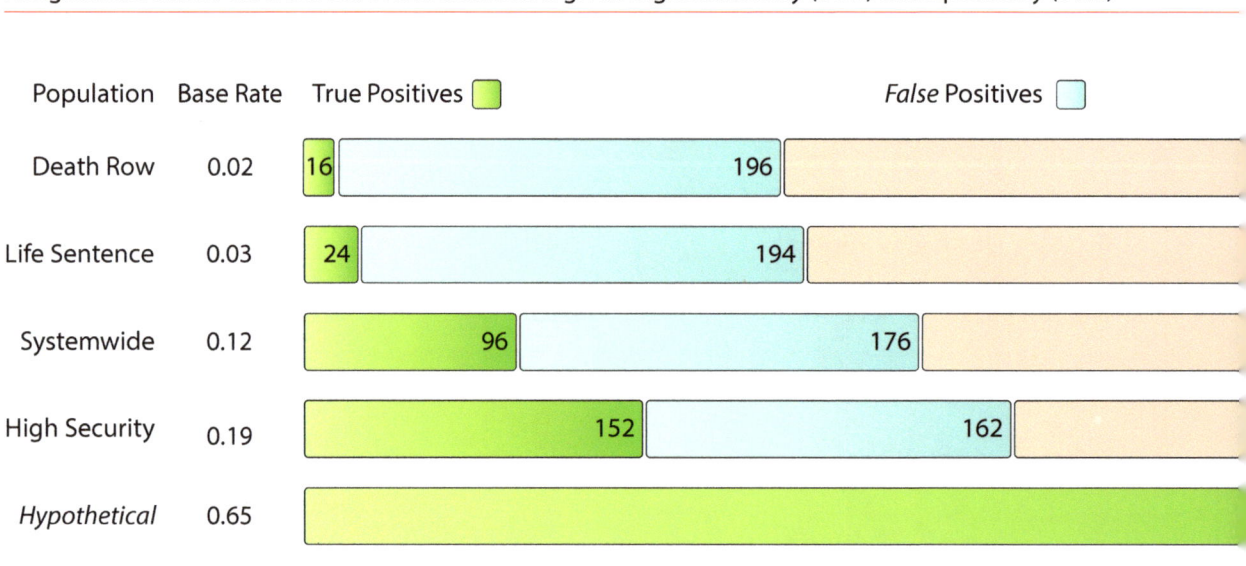

Assignments under different Base Rate conditions given high Sensitivity (80%) and Specificity (80%)

As seen in Figure 3[1], the 80% 'hit rate' for sensitivity and specificity ascribed to the hypothetical risk assessment tool is maintained across all of the base rates outlined, with correct assignment of risk remaining at 80% and the combined rate of false positives and false negatives remaining at 20%.

In a clinical context, however, the 20% 'error margin' is of substantive significance. Whilst sensitivity and specificity remain invariant, in absolute terms the incidence of 'false positives' becomes increasingly unacceptable as base rates tend towards lower values and the incidence of 'false negatives' becomes increasingly unacceptable as base rates tend towards higher values. Comparing the most extreme values at the lowest base rate of 0.02, one would have to accept the risk of misclassifying 196 individuals as being at risk of violence in order to correctly identify 16 individuals actually at risk of violence. What's more, this difficult decision would still leave 4 violent individuals misclassified as non-violent. At the (hypothetical) highest base rate of 0.65, the problem is transposed, but still exists. At this base rate, 130 people at risk of violence would be misclassified as *not* being at risk of violence.

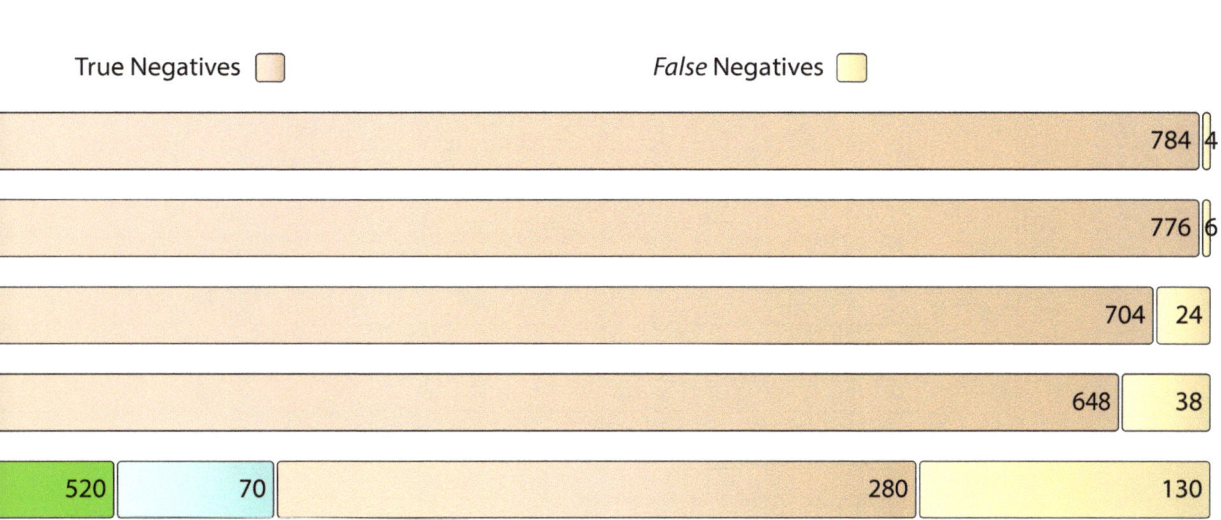

1	Note here that values have been set per 1000 to clarify the distinctions between columns. The actual N per group in Cunningham and Reidy's study was 100. An hypothetical population with a high base rate has been added for comparative purposes.

To give the above issue a meaningful clinical context, Wollert (2006) has estimated actual values for the sensitivity and specificity of a number of commonly used actuarial tools using populations with known base rates for sex offending. The tools used in this study were:

- Minnesota Sex Offender Screening Tool – Revised (MnSOST-R Epperson, Kaul and Hessleton 1999)

- Rapid Risk Assessment for Sex Offender Recidivism (RRASOR) Hanson 1997

- Sex Offender Risk Appraisal Guide (SORAG Quinsey, Harris, Rice & Cormier 1998)

- Static-99 (Hanson & Thornton 2000)

- Violence Risk Appraisal Guide (VRAG GT Harris et al 1993)

Figure 4

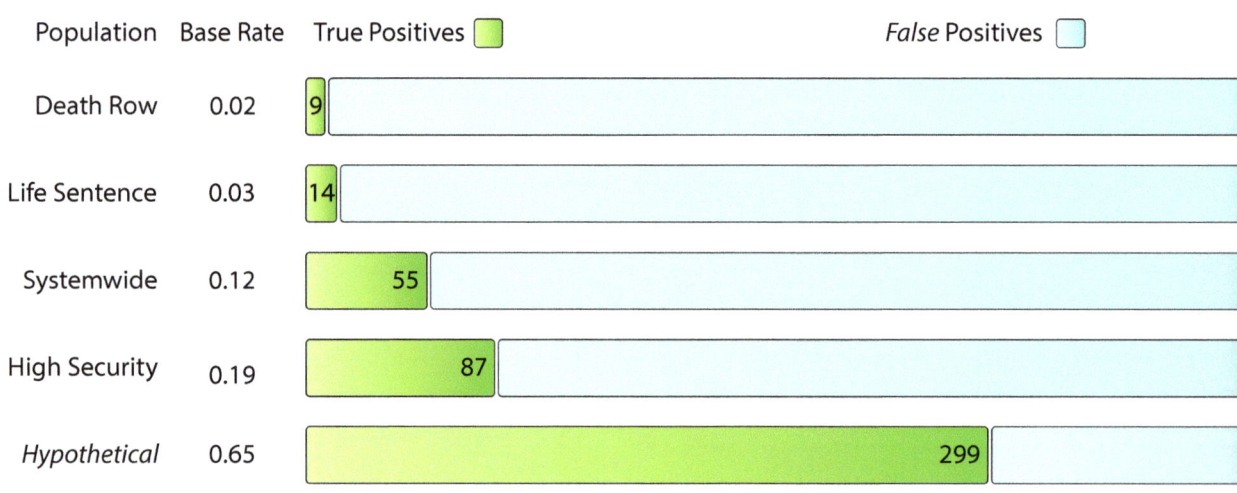

All of the above tools have been shown by one or more studies to have reasonable psychometric properties (reliability and validity for the majority and reliability, validity and discriminatory power in the case of the VRAG). Underlining the point that these measures are not the most pertinent to clinical practice, Wollert estimated in contrast that the highest sensitivity and specificity for the above tools was 0.46 and 0.15 respectively, with the average ratio of sensitivity to specificity (a measure of the divergence between the two measures) lying at around 0.33. Note here, that Wollert evaluated the tools not only against the prediction of immediate or short term violence, but also rated their predictive abilities over fairly long timescales. No improvement in outcomes was noted. Keying these 'real world' values into the previous Figure gives the values set out in Figure 4[2].

It can be seen from Figure 4 that once 'real world' values for sensitivity and specificity are considered, the absolute 'error margin' attributable to risk assessment becomes even less palatable than that outlined for the idealised scenario in Figure 3. Looking again at the more extreme ends of the spectrum for sensitivity and specificity, in a 'Death Row' population of 1,000, one would have to accept the misclassification of 833 people as likely to be violent in order to correctly identify 9 people as being at risk of violence. This would then still leave the majority of people actually at risk of being violent (N=11) misclassified as *not* at risk of violence.

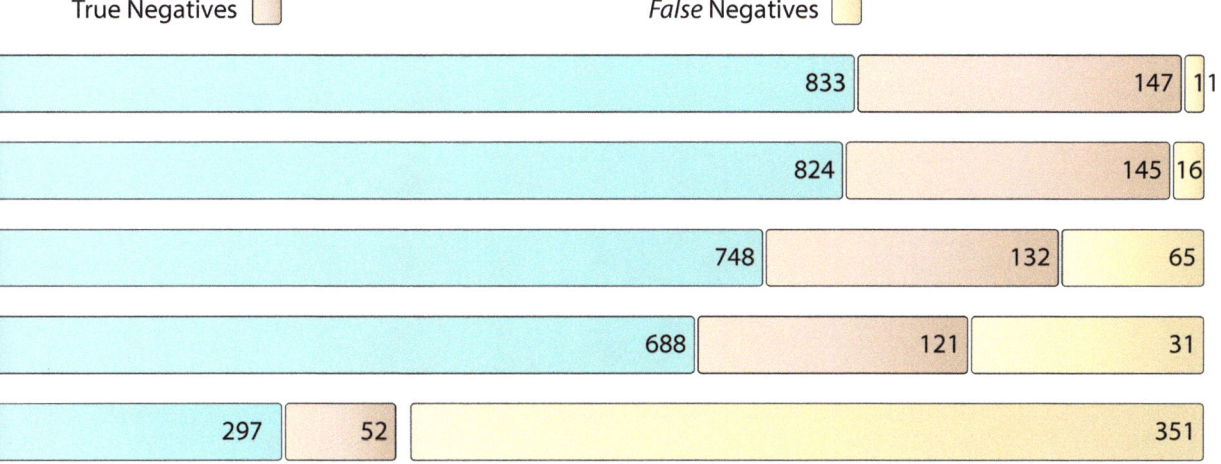

[2] Where numbers in this Figure do not sum to exactly 1000 this is due to rounding.

Conversely, at the highest (hypothetical) base rate considered, the 'average' risk assessment tool evaluated in Wollert's study, would misclassify 351 people who were at risk of violence as not being at such risk.

Wollert concludes that "actuarials are useless for identifying likely sexual recidivists from populations with recidivism base rates below 0.25". He underlines the importance of bringing harsh statistical fact into the policy arena, making the challenging statement that "policy makers should acquaint themselves with Bayes' theorem so that they can understand why it is difficult to predict alarming but infrequent crimes with any reasonable degree of certainty, no matter how much money is spent….They can then explain this unpleasant reality to anxious constituents". The stark points made by Wollert regarding risk assessment are readily underlined by evidence from the Criminal Justice System. For example, the fact that prior to the advent of DNA testing, a substantial number of defendants charged with sex offences were falsely convicted (Gross et al 2005).

Notwithstanding the difficulties, the current reality of clinical practice is that decisions regarding risk have to be made. Acknowledging the base rate issues outlined above, there are essentially two options open to the clinician who needs to find a way of identifying a risk assessment tool providing the best available predictive balance. The first option is to find a comparative statistic which is independent of base rate but provides the type of 'overall estimate' apparently offered by the accuracy statistics. The second option is to acknowledge the reality of base rate-dependent variation and to evaluate risk assessment tools based on the perceived relative importance of the two forms of misclassification.

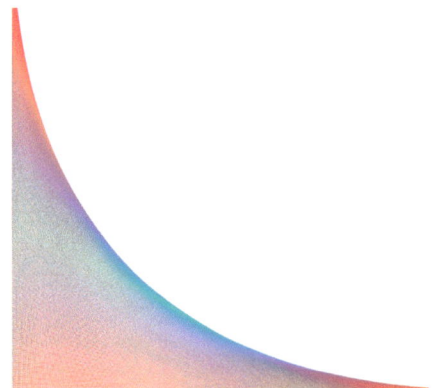

Receiver Operating curves (ROC curves) are one means commonly used to provide a single figure balancing sensitivity and specificity. ROC curves are graphs which plot values for sensitivity against (1-specificity). The area under the ROC curve (the AUC) provides a single figure, with an AUC of 0.5 indicating that the overall performance of the risk assessment tool is no better than chance, whilst an AUC of 1.0 implies perfect accuracy. The single figure is appealing and ROC curves are neutral to base rate (albeit only in the same statistical way that sensitivity and specificity are neutral to base rate). This is simply because the ROC is a visual representation of the space between sensitivity and specificity. The single figure provided by the AUC conveys no additional information to that available from considering sensitivity and specificity individually, it just makes the balance between sensitivity and specificity easier to interpret. It should be noted that the apparent objectivity of the single figure is also illusory. The area under the curve in practice defines a range of decision thresholds which represent the compromise between specificity and sensitivity. Clinicians using the ROC curve ultimately still have to make a subjective judgement regarding the relative importance of sensitivity and specificity. Comparing multiple risk assessment tools using ROC curves can be useful since it provides a visually accessible way of weighing up their relative merits. One risk tool may be more sensitive to identifying those at risk, another tool may be better at identifying those not at risk. Such benefits aside, ROC curves ultimately provide only the same information as considering sensitivity and specificity individually.

Considering alternative options for weighing the attributes of risk assessment tools, Kraemer (1987) has made the reasonable point that attempting to identify base-rate independent statistics is "a form of avoidance". Along similar lines, Uebersax (1987) has reasoned that to "really solve the base rate problem, it may be necessary to measure agreement on presence and absence of a disorder separately". Both approaches make the point that acknowledging the impact of base rate differentials may be of greater clinical significance than finding ways to (statistically) neutralise this impact for ease of interpretation. A second option open to clinicians then is to consider using statistics which explicitly identify confidence in the identification of true positives and true negatives at different base rates.

The statistics most commonly used in taking the above approach are **positive predictive value** and **negative predictive value**. Both are easily calculated from the contingency table outlined earlier following the formulae below:

Positive Predictive Value (PPV) = N of True Positives / (N of True Positives + N of False Positives)

Negative Predictive Value (NPV) = N of True Negatives / (N of True Negatives + N of False Negatives)

From these equations, it can be seen that positive predictive value (PPV) indicates the ratio of true positives to all identified positives, both correct and incorrect, whilst negative predictive value (NPV) indicates the ratio of true negatives to all identified negatives, both correct and incorrect. So, the positive predictive value of a risk tool indicates the confidence the clinician can have in the tool's ability to identify people who are at risk of being violent. The negative predictive value indicates the confidence the clinician can have in the tool's ability to identify people who are not at risk of being violent.

It is important to understand the quite distinct types of information which sensitivity and specificity versus positive and negative predictive value convey. The two sets of measures are often confused. The key to interpretation, as suggested above, lies in their differential association with population base rates. A risk assessment tool with a very high sensitivity can have a very low precision when there are far more true positives in the population than true negatives. Conversely, a risk assessment tool with a very high specificity can have low precision when there are far more true negatives than positives in the population.

Figure 5

Positive and negative predictive values based on actual estimates (assuming 46% Sensitivity and 15% Specificity)

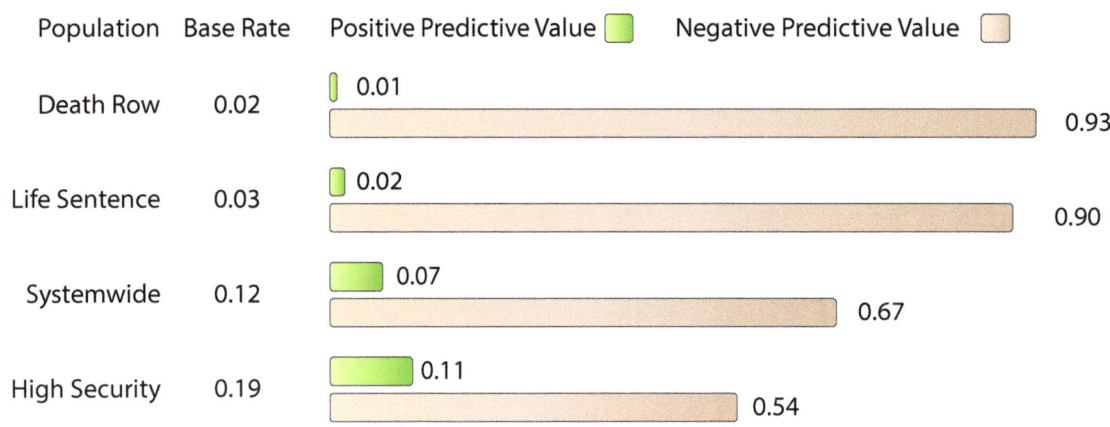

To provide a working example of how this distinction operates, Figure 5 above summarises the positive and negative predictive values which obtain across a range of base rates. As previously, the base rates chosen and the values set for sensitivity and specificity are taken from the 'real life' figures outlined earlier. Unlike measures of sensitivity and specificity, drawn from the same contingency table, the positive predictive value of the 'average' risk tool can be seen to increase with increasing base rate, whilst the negative predictive value of the risk assessment tool decreases. So, the values of PPV and NPV for a risk assessment tool provide clinicians with an insightful measure into their likely precision in the context of diverse base rates. This is much closer to the form of information which is most useful in clinical decision making. Note, however, that at low base rates such as those outlined here, it will always be easier to predict negatives than positives (and vice versa at high base rates).

Given the different forms of information conveyed by the range of statistics available for interpretation from a simple 2x2 contingency table alone, it would be of considerable benefit to clinicians if test manuals and the research literature provided a broader range of key statistics alongside the basic psychometric properties of actuarial tools. Arguably, the table of values allowing clinicians to get the best feel for the overall value of a risk assessment tool would set out:

- characteristics of the reference population using which the tool was developed

- sensitivity and specificity (indicating predictive power all else being equal)

- positive and negative predictive values for distinct base rates (indicating relative precision)

As a final note regarding the options open to clinicians in weighing the benefits of actuarial tools, it is worth putting the above information together to establish the base rates of violence at which actuarial prediction is likely to provide clinicians with a better than chance estimate of risk. In the following, Figure 6 summarises the required base rates for estimates of accuracy, positive predictive value and negative predictive value given Wollert's 'real world' estimates of sensitivity and specificity for common actuarial tools. Figure 7 gives these estimates based on idealised hypothetical tools with, respectively, very high sensitivity and very high specificity.

In the 'real world' scenario, it is again clear that overall accuracy is unlikely to be a particularly useful measure. Even at fairly extreme base rates (both low and high) the accuracy statistic fails to achieve a greater than chance prediction of violence/non-violence. What is slightly more disturbing, however, is that, given Wollert's plausible values for the likely sensitivity and specificity of the 'average' commonly used risk assessment tool, PPV and NPV require fairly extreme high and low base rates, respectively, for risk tools to achieve greater than chance estimates. At the extreme base rates suggested, it is not wholly unreasonable to say that tossing a coin might be as indicative of the actual risk of violence.

Of course, individual risk assessment tools may achieve higher levels of either sensitivity or specificity than the tools evaluated by Wollert. Equally, the tools evaluated by Wollert may achieve greater specificity and sensitivity in different reference populations or with a focus on different types of violence. Varying sensitivity and specificity to explore a more 'idealised' scenario however, the values in Figure 7 indicate a slightly disappointing outcome even for hypothetical risk assessment tools with high values of sensitivity or specificity. Whichever statistic is used (accuracy, PPV, NPV) population base rates need to be around the 50% mark for such risk assessment tools to achieve their goal of identifying people with or without the risk of violence at a greater than chance level.

Figure 6

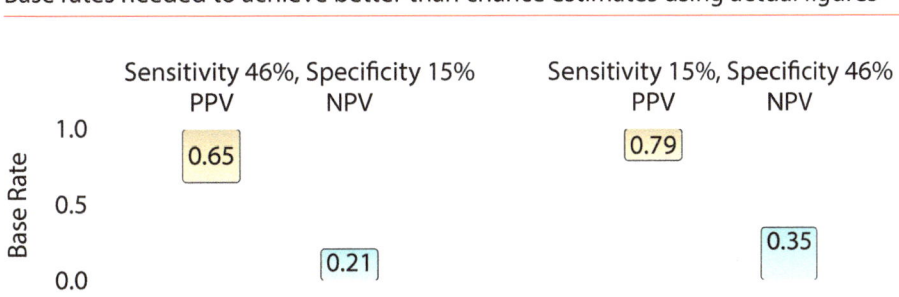

Base rates needed to achieve better than chance estimates using actual figures

Can these figures be improved on? If not, perhaps this is "what all the fuss is about" in respect of actuarial assessment (cf. Maden 2003)? Revisiting Figure 7, if both sensitivity and specificity are set to equivalent very high or very low values, accuracy simply tracks their joint value, regardless of base rate. However, 'above chance' values for PPV and NPV do improve in respect of the base rates needed for accurate assessment. Take the case of an assessment tool with 80% sensitivity and 80% specificity. In this instance, above chance values for PPV occur at population base rates of 21% and above, whilst above chance values for NPV occur at a base rate of 79% or below. Unfortunately, these base rates are still implausibly extreme for many forms of violence in many populations. Furthermore, it is also highly unlikely that any single risk assessment tool would achieve such high values for both sensitivity and specificity. There is invariably a trade-off between the two.

There are then problems with the base rate of violence which appear fairly intransigent. Given that clinicians are faced with engaging in risk assessment in populations with very low base rates (e.g. community rates for lethal violence) and with very high base rates (e.g. verbal aggression in secure wards) how can we improve on actuarial risk 'statistics' in future? One option would be to use 'split half' tools. That is, tools which address directly both sensitivity and specificity by including both empirically established risk factors and empirically established protective factors. A second option (cf. Monahan 1981) is to individualize risk assessment around the base rates. That is, to use the population base rate and associated actuarial risk assessment value as a starting point, from which an individual risk profile is developed by incorporating into the picture an individual's past aggressive behaviour and other dispositional (and situational) characteristics.

Figure 7

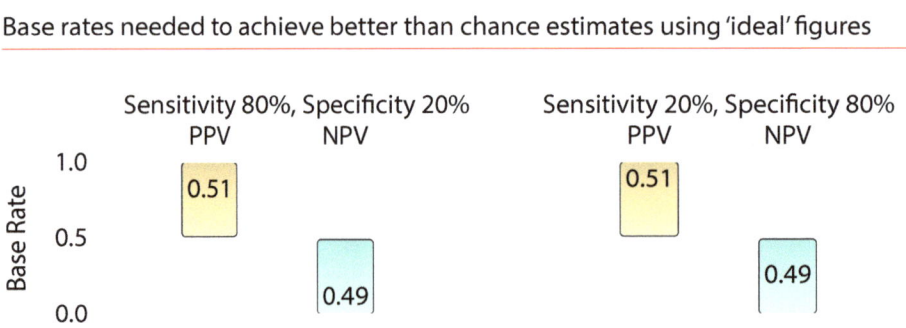

Is this a viable option? As Monahan states, the process of individualization should be undertaken conservatively and "only when reliable indicators are present that the individual differs significantly from the comparison group". Using pure clinical judgement to achieve individualization, however, would seem to render null and void the point of using actuarial assessment in the first place. As Maden (2003) has argued, the value of actuarial assessment over clinical judgement is that it is structured, reliable (or, at least, objective) and, perhaps most importantly, transparent.

To maintain the required level of transparency, the 'individualization' process could, alternatively, be achieved using statistical weightings in respect of factors known to influence the base rate of violence (e.g. gender, age, previous violent behaviour). However, transferring such weightings to the individual situation would make for relatively complex calculations and would also be of dubious statistical merit. The apparently 'objective' weightings would in reality only reflect the 'average' values achieved within a population, rather than values actually attributable to the individual.

Kraemer (1987) suggests a third option. She follows a 'signal to noise ratio' model, arguing that to achieve a high signal (true values) to noise (false values) ratio, either the signal needs to be amplified or the noise attenuated. In the context of risk assessment she suggests, signal 'amplification' would involve such strategies as multiple or consensus risk assessment, the development of better risk assessment tools and so on. Attenuating the noise would involve such approaches as better training, better standardization of risk tools and/or risk assessment 'test conditions' and better pre-screening of clients. The latter option (pre-screening) may be of value, in that such screening could partition out groups of clients in which the true base rate of violence is likely to be suitably high (or low) to allow risk assessment tools to perform well in respect of either sensitivity or specificity. It remains a moot point whether such screening in fact achieves the goal of improving actuarial risk prediction, or whether it simply creates a situation in which 'coin tossing' is likely to produce good results. Other options for signal enhancement/noise reduction would only be likely to offer enhanced sensitivity and specificity as base rates diverge significantly from 50%, leaving the problem that the clinician could only achieve one of two equally desirable outcomes (reduced false positives or reduced false negatives).

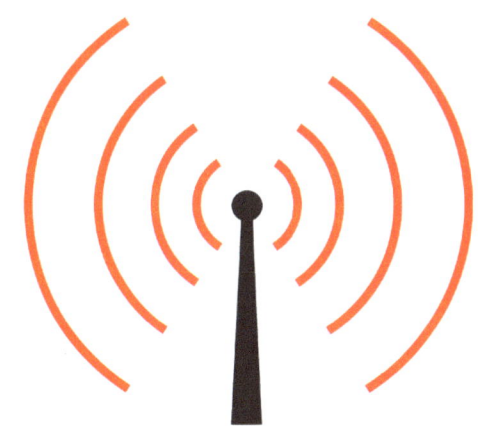

The above implies the rather dispiriting conclusion that we should perhaps abandon actuarial (and indeed any other form of risk assessment) in populations and sub-populations with 'problematic' base rates. Cicchetti et al (1991) argue instead that we should consider more carefully how to structure the evaluation of risk assessment tools within target populations. The argument is that since we can identify base rates within populations and sub-populations prior to making the attempt to evaluate a tool, we can also identify in advance the sample sizes needed to make the attempt at evaluation a meaningful one. Cicchetti suggests a rule of thumb of at least 10 actual positive cases in the reference sample population (or sub-population). So, where the prevalence of the violent behaviour in question is 5% in a particular population, an appropriate reference sample would need to comprise a minimum of 200 individuals. Where the base rate decreases to 1%, 1000 individuals would be needed.

Given that the median sample size for studies evaluating actuarial risk assessment tools is currently around 151 (cf. Leitner et al 2006), it is clear that we have some way to go in following the optimal design strategy suggested by Cicchetti. It is nonetheless a worthy goal and the numbers needed may be achieved via better collaboration between researchers and clinicians. As with many aspects of violence risk assessment and management greater transparency and a stronger co-operative bond between clinicians, researchers and policy makers would be of great benefit. Whether newer generations of risk assessment tool will utilise better strategies for evaluation and better methods of communicating the realisable potential for precise risk assessment remains to be seen.

Base rates: the 'cognitive' problem

The above outlined issues relate to the understanding and interpretation of statistical data. As noted, the 'base rate problem' also has an aspect which is more cognitive than statistical. This is to do with the fact that whilst people, subconsciously, use base rates to make probability judgements on a routine basis (Koehler 1966) they often struggle with the correct interpretation of probability. This cognitive problem can also be transposed as a problem of communication (Dvoskin & Heilbrun 2001). There are many ways of communicating risk, but even assuming that these are relevant, empirically supported and applicable to a clinical population, risk communicated in a way that is not understood by the clinician will have little merit in helping with accurate assessment.

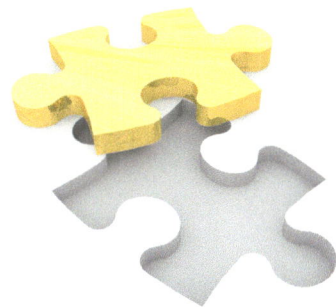

As the cognitive 'base rate fallacy' (cf. Manis 1980) is not an intrinsic function of base rates, but rather a problem relating to how people process information, the issue will only be touched on briefly here. It serves to provide further context in relation to the problems which may arise in the clinical setting when actuarial data are used for individual-level risk assessment. An in-depth overview of the cognitive problems encountered in the interpretation of probability is given in Martins (2006). Interestingly, Martins concludes that such errors are the inevitable consequence of humans following an innate but flawed Bayesian heuristic. Whatever the cause, the main failures in judgements of probability which have been identified are as follows:

- Base rate neglect (Kahneman & Tversky 1973; Bar-Hillel 1980)

- Overestimation of the probability of conjoined events (Cohen et al 1979)

- Failure to observe correlations within a pattern of events (Chapman & Chapman 1967)

- Attribution of causal correlations where events simply happen to co-occur (Chapman & Chapman 1967)

It can readily be seen how each of the above errors in probability judgement might apply to the assessment of individual risk in the clinical setting. For the purposes of the current guide, the most relevant error is base rate neglect. This is the tendency to ignore base rate information in favour of individuating information which the assessor perceives as of higher salience (Bar-Hillel 1980). In effect, the assessor (the clinician in this context) generates intuitive observations regarding characteristics of the client being assessed and these are given a greater cognitive weighting than specific and relevant knowledge regarding the characteristics of the (clinical) group to which the client belongs. This error perhaps explains the pressure to move from unstructured clinical assessment to actuarial assessment. It is possible that further research in the field of 'flawed cognition' will allow us to move to a point where we can usefully integrate clinical and actuarial risk assessment.

Summary and key points

Violence in the UK remains a significant public health issue and clinicians have inherited a substantive burden of responsibility for ensuring that effective risk assessment is carried out. Significant problems with the accuracy of unstructured clinical decision making paved the way for a new generation of risk assessment tool based on psychometric principles. These actuarial tools have been demonstrated to improve the accuracy of risk assessment beyond that of clinical judgement alone, but present their own problems in respect of interpreting outcomes. One of the major challenges for clinicians using these tools, lies in the meaningful transfer of statistical information produced in a reference population to a setting in which outcomes for an individual client are the main focus. The clinician needs at least a 'best guess' mechanism for evaluating the confidence they should have in the range of actuarial tools available to them.

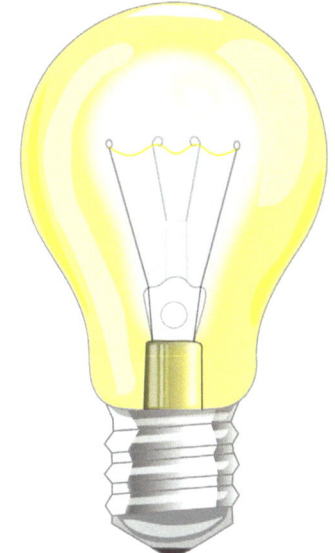

The statistics presented in the research literature and often also in the test manuals for the wide range of available actuarial tools is unhelpful, in that it generally focuses on the basic psychometric properties of reliability and validity. These statistics provide the clinician only with a measure of confidence in the coherence of the risk tool, not in its ability to predict relevant outcomes for the individual client. Short of evaluating a risk tool for each client individually, this ideal state will never be achieved. However, for tools used to categorise individuals into a small number of discrete risk categories, basic contingency tables drawn from reference population profiles can provide some insight into likely predictive value.

One key issue which can hamper the interpretation of such profiles is the so called 'base rate problem'. To reiterate a point made in the main text, this problem is actually a composite of three issues:

- The dependence of an assessment tool's accuracy on base rates in reference and target populations

- Limitations on predictive values (sensitivity, specificity and related statistics) for rare behaviours

- Cognitive 'misinterpretation' of probabilistic information

Using a number of worked examples, this guide has explored the base rate problem from a clinical perspective, using both 'idealised' and 'real world' values for actuarial risk assessment tools. The worked examples have highlighted a number of points the clinician needs to be aware of in interpreting the confidence with which evaluations of actuarial tools in reference populations can be transposed into assumptions regarding the likely value of the tool(s) for a given clinical population.

Given the importance of accurate risk assessment and the lack of exposure commonly offered to clinicians and other professionals in respect of the statistical niceties of risk prediction, the main goal of this guide has been to provide a pragmatic primer for 'real world' risk assessment. The key points can be summarised as follows:

- Predictive values achieved for a tool in a reference population are only applicable to clinical populations with the same or at least a broadly similar structure

- The sensitivity and specificity of a risk assessment tool are independent of population size and independent of the base rate of violence in that population

- Overall accuracy (a single figure balance between sensitivity and specificity) is strongly dependent on base rate

- Where sensitivity and specificity are *equivalent* for a risk tool overall accuracy provides no additional information

- Where sensitivity and specificity *diverge*, overall accuracy tends towards values for sensitivity at high base rates of violence and towards specificity at low base rates of violence

- For the above reasons, overall accuracy gives a misleading impression of the likely predictive value of a risk assessment tool

- Low base rates of violence result in unpalatable absolute error margins, even where a risk assessment tool has a genuinely high predictive value

- Estimates suggest that base rates below 25% (a common value in many clinical settings) produce actuarial predictions which are little better than chance

- By calculating the positive predictive value and negative predictive value of a risk tool, it is possible to accurately identify the degree of confidence one can have in the predictive value of that tool at different base rates

- Potentially 'innate' cognitive difficulties in the correct interpretation of probabilistic data further hamper the goal of the clinician in determining the likely risk of violence in individual clients and client groups

- Ongoing research to provide more sophisticated approaches to risk assessment and to untangle the issues raised by cognitive dissonance in the interpretation of probabilistic information may help to promote more accurate risk assessment in the future

Whilst waiting for future developments in the research literature, we need a strategy to improve clinical confidence in the value of available risk assessment tools. Accurate and informative comparisons between available risk assessment tools can be promoted by a more rigorous approach to the evaluation of such tools.

One key advance which could be made in this context, is the use of adequate reference sample sizes. Equally, however, the interpretation of predictive value needs to be made more meaningful for clinicians. Here, we can improve on the current situation by ensuring that relevant statistics for reference and clinical populations are made readily available, both in test manuals and more widely. Appropriate training may also need to be put in place to ensure that clinicians become comfortable with and skilled in the routine use of such statistics.

References and further reading

Alberg, A.J., Wan Park, J., Brant, M.P.H. et al (2004) *The use of 'overall accuracy' to evaluate the validity of screening or diagnostic tests* Journal of General Internal Medicine 19: 460-465

Bar-Hillel, M. (1980) *The base rate fallacy in probability judgements* Acta Psychologica 44 211-233

Baxstrom vs. Herald (1966) 383 US 107

Boer, D.P., Hart, S.D., Kropp, P.R. et al (1997) *Manual for the Sexual Violence Risk-20: Professional Guidelines for Assessing Risk of Sexual Violence.* Vancouver, B.C.: British Columbia Institute on Family Violence

Chapman, L.J., & Chapman, J. P. (1967). *Genesis of popular but erroneous psychodiagnostic observations.* Journal of Abnormal Psychology, 72, 193-204.

Cicchetti, D.V. (1991) *Establishing the reliability and validity of neuropsychological disorders with low base rates: Some recommended guidelines* Journal of Clinical and Experimental Neuropsychology 13:2 328-338

Cohen, J., Chesnick, E.I., & Haran, D., (1979). *Evaluation of compound probabilities in sequential choice.* Nature 232, 414-416.

Cunningham, M.D. & Reidy, T.J. (1998) *Integrating base rate data in violence risk assessments at capital sentencing* Behavioural Sciences and the Law 16: 71-95

Dix, G.E. (1976) *Differential processing of abnormal sex offenders: Utilization of California's Mentally Disordered Sex Offender Program* Journal of Criminal Law and Criminology 67: 233-243

Dolan, M. & Doyle, M. (2000) *Violence Risk Prediction: Clinical and actuarial measures and the role of the Psychopathy Checklist* British Journal of Psychiatry 177: 303-311

Epperson, D., Kaul, J. & Heeselton, D. (1999) *Minnesota Sex Offender Screening Tool – Revised (MnSOST-R) Development, performance and recommended risk level cut scores* Unpublished Manuscript

Fuller, J. & Cowan, J. (1999) *Risk assessment in a multi-disciplinary forensic setting: Clinical judgement revisited.* Journal of Forensic Psychiatry 10: 276-289

Gardner, W., Lidz, C.W., Mulvey, E.P. et al (1996) *A comparison of actuarial methods for identifying repetitively violent patients with mental illnesses.* Law and Human Behaviour 20: 35-48

Glaros, A.G. & Kline, R.B. (1988) *Understanding the accuracy of tests with cutting scores: The sensitivity, specificity and predictive value model.* Journal of Clinical Psychology 44: 6 1013-1023

Gross, S.R., Jacoby, K., Matheson, D. et al (2005) *Exonerations in the United States 1989 through 2003* Journal of Criminal Law and Criminology 95: 523-561

Hall, G.C.N. (1988) *Criminal behaviour as a function of clinical and actuarial variables in a sex offender population* Journal of Consulting and Clinical Psychology 56 773-775

Hanson, R.K. (1997) *The development of a brief actuarial risk scale for sexual offense recidivism*. Unpublished Manuscript

Hanson, R.K. & Thornton, D. (2000) *Improving risk assessments for sex offenders: A comparison of three actuarial scales*. Law and Human Behaviour 24: 119-136

Hare, R.D. (1991) *Manual for the Hare Psychopathy Checklist-Revised*. Toronto, Canada: Multi-Health Systems

Harris, G.T., Rice, M.E. & Quinsey, V. L. (1993) *Violent recidivism of mentally disordered offenders: The development of a statistical prediction instrument*. Criminal Justice and Behaviour 20: 315-335

Hart, S.D. (1998a) *Psychopathy and risk for violence*. In: Psychopathy: Theory, research and implications for Society (Eds. D. Cooke, A.E. Forth & R. Hare) 355-375 Dordrecht, The Nerherlands: Kluwer

Hirschi, T. & Gottfredson, M. (1989) *Age and the explanation of crime*. American Journal of Sociology 89: 552-584

Kahn, T.J. & Chambers, H. (1991) *Assessing reoffense risk with juvenile sex offenders* Child Welfare 70: 333-345

Kahneman, D. & Tversky, A. (1973) *On the psychology of prediction* Psychological Review 80: 237-251

Koehler, J.J. (1996) *The base rate fallacy reconsidered: Descriptive, normative and methodological challenges*. Behavioural and Brain Sciences 19: 1-59

Kraemer, H.C. (1982) *Estimating false alarms and missed events from inter-observor agreement: Comment on Kaye*. Psychological Bulletin 92: 749-754

Kraemer, H.C. (1987) *Charlie Brown and Statistics: An Exchange* Archives of General Psychiatry 44: 192-193

Kropp, P.R., Hart, S.D., Webster, C.W. et al (1995) *Manual for the Spousal Assault Risk Assessment Guide, 2nd Edition*. Vancouver, BC: British Columbia Institute on Family Violence

Leitner, M., Barr, W., McGuire, J., Jones, S. & Whittington, R. (2006) *Systematic review of prevention and intervention strategies for populations at high risk of engaging in violent behaviour: Final report*. University of Liverpool, Liverpool/InfotechUK Research Ltd, Cheshire, UK (507 pages).

Lidz, C.W., Mulvey, E.P. & Gardner, W. (1993) *The accuracy of predictions of violence to others*. Journal of the American Medical Association 269: 1007-1111

Maden, A. (2003) *Standardised risk assessment: Why all the fuss?* Psychiatric Bulletin 27: 201-204

Manis, M., Dovalina, I., Avis, N.E. & Cardoze, S. (1980) *Base rates can affect individual predictions* Journal of Personality and Social Psychology 63: 231-248

Martins, A.C.R. (2006) *Probability biases as Bayesian inference* Judgement and Decision Making 1:2 108-117

Metz, C.E. (1978) *Basic principles of ROC analysis* Seminars in Nuclear Medicine Vol. VIII 4: 283-298

Miller, S.J., Dinitz, S. & Conrad, J.P. (1982) *Careers of the violent: The dangerous offender and criminal justice* Lexington, MA: Lexington Books

Monahan, J. (1981) *Predicting violent behaviour: An assessment of clinical techniques.* Beverley Hills: Sage

Monahan, J. & Steadman, H.J. (1994, Eds.) *Violence and Mental Disorder: Developments in Risk Assessment* Chicago, Ill.: University of Chicago Press

Monahan, J., Steadman, H.J. Clark Robbins, P. et al (2005) *An actuarial model of violence risk assessment for persons with mental disorder* Psychiatric Services 56:7 810-815

Morris, N. & Miller, M. (1985) *Predictions of dangerousness.* In: M. Tonry & N. Morris (Eds.) Crime and Justice: An Annual Review of Research (Vol. 6) 1-50 Chicago: Chicago University Press

Mossman, D. (1994) *Assessing predictions of violence: Being accurate about accuracy.* Journal of Consulting and Clinical Psychology 62: 783-792

Mulvey, E.P. & Lidz, C.W. (1985) *Back to Basics: A critical analysis of dangerousness research in a new legal environment.* Law and Human Behaviour 9: 209-219

Nisbett, R.E., Borgida, E. Crandall, R. & Reed, H. (1976) *Popular induction: Information is not always informative.* In: J.S. Carroll & J.W. Payne (Eds.) Cognition and social behaviour 2: 227-236

Quinsey, V.L., Harris, G., Rice, M. & Cornier, C. (1998) *Violent Offenders* Washington, DC: American Psychological Association

Royal College of Psychiatrists (2005) *National Audit of Violence and Aggression* London:RCP

Saari, R.J. & Saari, L. (2002) *Actuarial risk assessment with elderly sex offenders: Should it be abandoned?* Sex Offender Law Report 3(5) 68: 73-76

Serin, R.C. & Amos, N.L. (1995) *The role of psychopathy in the assessment of dangerousness.* International Journal of Law and Psychiatry 18: 231-238

Shapiro, D.E. (1999) *The interpretation of diagnostic tests.* Statistical Methods in Medical Research 8: 113-34

Shlonsky, A. & Wagner, D. (2005) *The next step: Integrating actuarial risk assessment and clinical judgement into an evidence-based practice framework in CPS case management* Children and Youth Services Review 27:4 409-427

Shrout, P.E., Spitzer, R.L. & Fleiss, J.L. (1987) *Quantification of agreement in psychiatric diagnosis revisited* Archives of General Psychiatry 44: 172-177

Smith, S.M. (1993) *The prediction of dangerous behaviour.* In: P.J. Resnick (Ed.) Forensic Psychiatry Review Course American Academy of Psychiatry and the Law 539-541

Snowden, P. (1997) *Practical aspects of clinical risk assessment and management.* British Journal of Psychiatry 170 (suppl. 32): 32-34

Steadman, H.J. & Coccoza, J.J. (1974) *Careers of the Criminally Insane : Excessive Social Control of Deviance* Lexington, MA: Lexington Books

Swanson, J.W., Holzer, C.E. III, Granju, V.K. & Jono, R.T. (1990) *Violence and psychiatric disorder in the community: Evidence from the epidemiologic catchment area surveys* Hospital and Community Psychiatry 41: 761-770

Szklo, M. & Nieto, F.J. *Epidemiology: Beyond the basics* Gaithersburg, MD:Aspen Publishers Inc.

Szmukler, G. (2001) *Violence risk prediction in practice.* British Journal of Psychiatry 178: 84-85

Szmukler, G. (2003) *Risk assessment: 'numbers' and 'values'* Psychiatric Bulletin 27: 205-207

Tarasoff vs. Regents of the University of California (1976).

Uebersax, J.S. (1987) *Letter to the Editor* Archives of General Psychiatry 44: 193-194

Walker, A., Flatley, J., Kershaw, C. & Moon, D. (2009) *Crime in England and Wales 2008/2009 Volume 1: Findings from the British Crime Survey and Police Recorded Crime* London: Home Office Statistical Bulletin 11/09 Volume 1

Webster, C.D., Douglas, K.S., Eaves, D. et al (1997a) *Assessing risk of violence to others.* In Impulsivity: Theory, Assessment and Treatment (Eds. C.D. Webster & M.A. Jackson, New York: Guilford Press)

Webster, C.D., Douglas, K.S., Eaves, D. et al (1997b) *HCR-20: Assessing risk of violence (version 2)* Vancouver: Mental Health Law & Policy Institute, Simon Fraser University

Wollert, R. (2002) *The importance of cross-validation in actuarial test construction: Shrinkage in the risk estimates for the Minnesota Sex Offender Screening Tool - Revised* Journal of Threat Assessment 2(1): 87-102

Wollert, R. (2006) *Low base rates limit expert certainty when current actuarials are used to identify sexually violent predators: An application of Bayes' Theorem* Psychology, Public Policy and Law 12: 1 56-85

Index

A

accuracy 1, 2, 7, 10, 11, 12, 13, 14, 18, 21, 22, 28, 29, 31, 32, 33, 34
actuarial 1, 2, 3, 4, 5, 6, 7, 16, 21, 22, 23, 24, 25, 26, 27, 28, 29, 31, 32, 34, 35, 36
assault 1, 13

B

base rate 7, 9, 10, 11, 12, 13, 14, 15, 18, 19, 21, 22, 23, 24, 25, 26, 28, 29, 31, 33
  base rate fallacy 26, 31, 33
  base rate neglect 26
base rates 7, 9, 10, 11, 12, 13, 14, 15, 18, 19, 21, 22, 23, 24, 25, 26, 28, 29, 31, 33

C

chance 2, 18, 21, 22, 29
classification tree 2
classified 7
client 1, 3, 4, 5, 6, 7, 9, 27, 28, 30
  clients 1, 3, 5, 9, 24, 30
clinical assessment 2, 3, 27
  clinical decision making 3, 21, 28
  clinical evaluation 2
  clinical judgement 2, 5, 23, 28, 35
  clinical prediction 2, 3
clinical staff 1
  clinician 1, 3, 4, 5, 6, 7, 9, 10, 11, 18, 20, 24, 26, 28, 29, 30
  clinicians 1, 3, 4, 10, 19, 21, 23, 25, 28, 30
cognitive 7, 28
  cognitive problem 26
contingency 8, 10, 11, 19, 21, 28, 37
  contingency table 8, 10, 11, 19, 21, 37
  contingency tables 8, 28, 37
cut-off 6, 8

D

diagnostic 6, 11, 31, 35
discriminatory power 4, 5, 17
dynamic factors 3

E

error 15, 17, 26, 27, 29
estimates 8, 29
evaluation 2, 4, 7, 24, 25, 30
  evaluations 4, 29

F

false negatives 19
false positives 19
forensic 1, 32

H

harm 1

I

Incidence 7
interpretation 1, 7, 19, 20, 21, 26, 28, 30, 35

L

legal 1, 34
legal obligation 1
likelihood 4, 7, 10

M

measure 4, 5, 10, 12, 13, 17, 19, 21, 28
Mental Health Act 1
misclassification 18
model 6, 24, 32, 34

N

negative predictive value 19, 20, 21, 30

O

offender 3, 32, 34
outcome 2, 4, 5, 7, 22
  outcomes 1, 2, 3, 4, 6, 7, 8, 9, 10, 17, 24, 28

P

policy makers 18, 25
population 1, 4, 6, 7, 8, 9, 10, 11, 12, 15, 17, 20, 21, 22, 23, 24, 26, 28, 29, 32
practice 1, 3, 4, 12, 14, 17, 18, 19, 35, 36
prediction 2, 3, 4, 17, 21, 24, 32, 33, 35, 36
  positive predictive value 19, 20, 21, 30
  predicting 14
  predictive values 7, 20, 21, 28
  predictor 14
prevalence 6, 7, 13, 24
probability 26, 31
  probabilistic 7, 28, 30
psychometric 2, 4, 7, 17, 21, 28
public concern 1
public health 1, 28

R

raters 2, 4
receiver operating curves 18
reference population 4, 9, 10, 21, 28, 29
reliability 2, 4, 17, 28, 31
research 2, 3, 4, 5, 6, 21, 27, 28, 30, 33, 34
responsibility 1, 28
risk 1, 2, 3, 4, 6, 7, 9, 10, 11, 12, 13, 14, 15, 17, 18, 19, 20, 21, 22, 23, 24, 25, 26, 27, 28, 29, 30, 31, 32, 33, 34, 35, 36
  risk assessment 1, 2, 3, 4, 6, 7, 9, 10, 11, 12, 13, 14, 15, 17, 18, 19, 20, 21, 22, 23, 24, 25, 26, 27, 28, 29, 30, 33, 34, 35
  risk assessment tools 1, 2, 4, 7, 9, 10, 18, 19, 22, 24, 25, 29, 30
  risk items 2

S

sample size 25
sensitivity 6, 7, 9, 10, 11, 12, 13, 14, 15, 16, 17, 18, 19, 20, 21, 22, 23, 24, 28, 29, 32
signal to noise ratio 24
specificity 6, 7, 8, 9, 10, 11, 12, 13, 14, 15, 16, 17, 18, 19, 20, 21, 22, 23, 24, 28, 29, 32
statistics 5, 6, 7, 8, 9, 18, 19, 21, 23, 28, 30
  statistical 3, 4, 18, 24, 26, 28, 32
systematic review 4

T

Tarasoff 1, 36
target population 9, 10
true negatives 19
true positives 19

U

unstructured 2, 3, 5, 27, 28

V

validated 2, 4
validity 2, 4, 17, 28, 31
victim 3
  victims 1
victimisation 1
violence 1, 2, 3, 4, 6, 7, 9, 10, 11, 12, 15, 16, 17, 18, 21, 22, 23, 24, 25, 28, 29, 30, 31, 33, 34, 35, 36
violent 1, 2, 4, 6, 7, 8, 9, 10, 12, 15, 18, 20, 24, 32, 33, 34, 36

www.ingramcontent.com/pod-product-compliance
Lightning Source LLC
Chambersburg PA
CBHW050401180526
45159CB00005B/2102

9 781534 847767